Introduction

In order to get the very best that we can out of life, we must first endeavor to bring out the very best in ourselves. That entails applying a wholesome approach to our health in its entirety by encompassing not only its physical and nutritional components, but equally as important, its emotional, social and spiritual counterparts.

It is a well-known fact that if we are healthy and happy, the chances are we can live longer, better and higher quality lives. If we are spiritually resilient, we are able to make virtuous choices and deal with turmoil in a way that will benefit and not detract from our lives. If we are physically fit, we feel and look great and are more likely to have improved mental wellbeing.

This in turn, leads to us making better choices over what and how we eat, and how we live our lives. The one impacts the other and this book will guide you through an easy way to live a happy, healthy, fit and blessed life.

The Wholesome Life is a simple, hands-on book with useful and practical tips and advice set up as a day to day format for living a nourished, robust and content life.

Some of the ideas may be new to you, others may be useful to try and still, others may be challenging or life changing.

Let go of your inhibitions and give it a go!

It is my hope that this book can clearly set forth some modest guidelines for healthy living and thereby improve the quality of your life.

It goes without saying that as unique individuals we all have different physical abilities and mental, nutritional and spiritual requirements. Therefore, do not overexert yourself to the attainment of a suggestion. Do what is comfortable and realistic for you, always listening to your mind, spirit and body!

Please note that not all of the information in this book may be suitable for you to apply to your personal circumstances. Therefore, it is important to check with your doctor or medical care provider when changing your lifestyle.

Nevertheless, the information from this book may provide you with some basic guidelines for developing your own healthy living plan and regimen and as such living a wholesome, balanced and healthy life.

I welcome you to the start of this amazing journey.

Share the love!

In Health and Happiness,

Leanora

A Foreword

.... Before you begin The Wholesome Life....

My personal stance in life is one that entails, 'everything in moderation'. When you begin Day 1, you may feel a sudden urge to declutter, detox and get rid. There is no need to go and empty your cupboards and clear your home of every single thing devoid of nutrition, beauty, and inspiration (although at some point in the book you may feel the urge to) and by all means then do as you feel led to.

Make these changes daily. Make small amendments one day at a time. Take it day by day as you go through some of the very easy to apply suggestions in this book. Focus on starting where you can and from a point that causes you the least angst. This entire process should be uplifting.

This is your new standard of living. A happy, blessed, fit and active, nourished life! You can start from where you are right now and make significant changes that will positively impact your overall health. Commit to change and it will give you pleasing results.

This book is broken down into sections; 'happy, a bible verse, healthy, fit and an action'.

Happy: Each day make an effort to address the emotional barriers to your mental wellbeing. Whatever is detracting you from reaching your desired emotional state should be addressed. Seek to work with a counselor, mentor, pastor, homeopath, doctor, trusted friend or family member as you go through this book.

Maybe you are struggling with depression, anxiety, worry or you are still reliving a trauma that you have not healed from. Whatever it is, I encourage you to tackle these issues bravely, do not submerge them. There is no glory in submission. Face each area head on. Rise and blossom!

Yes, it may be difficult, yes you will have to address things that you have buried, BUT you will then also be able to come to terms with and understand why these things happened, the lesson you needed to learn and what to do going forward. Most importantly, after properly working through your issues, you can finally lay them to rest knowing that they will never be a source of anxiety, stress or upset again. Then you will have true freedom!

Remember, no one on this earth is perfect. We all have something we need to work on. It is my belief that those who conquer their demons are those who experience true freedom on this earth.

Learn to understand your own emotional states and figure out what best aids in getting you to a peaceful and content state of being. It may be that you find you are able to attain these states in music, prayer, meditation, aromatherapy, art, writing, in complete solitude, participating in a sport, working with animals, gardening, being actively social, or by practicing an alternative therapy.

Find out which method best suits your personality type. Be honest with yourself about your likes and your dislikes. There is no right or wrong. Here it is okay to be self-centered and wholly focused on your own personal gratification. There are no gray areas here. You either like something or you don't. It makes you happy or it does not. You feel calm after or you do not. We are all human, and as such, we are all beautifully flawed. We are all a work in progress. Take the time to explore different avenues. Search until you find the outlet that is note perfect for you. It should bring out your radiance and give you complete serenity and boundless bliss! Decide now that you deserve to be happy. Make it your t to be happy. Do what it takes for you to be happy.

Healthy: I am a strong believer that we should eat as humanely, naturally and as organically as possible. Therefore, I wholeheartedly encourage that we understand which foods we should be eating, for our body types, for their alkalizing, health promoting effects in our bodies and for their overall nutritional benefits to us.

In this book, there will be some suggestions pertaining to a variety of foods you can try. On your journey, only eat the foods that you like. Just because it is healthy does not mean you should suffer to eat it. Eat well and enjoy the process. Here are some tips to get you started:

- Focus on organic seeded fruits and vegetables (check out the clean fifteen and dirty dozen lists). This entails that the fruit and vegetables you consume should be pesticide free, void of wax (if it is not possible to find unwaxed fruit and vegetables, cleaning and soaking your fruit and vegetables in apple cider vinegar and/or baking soda should help to remove the wax), GMO-free and where possible locally grown (farmer's markets will have locally grown produce).

- Learn to make your own food. From homemade cakes and bread to soups and juices to a full on proper three-course meal. If it is home cooked, you can choose what goes in, what stays out and how it is prepared. Now if per chance, you are terrified of cooking for fear of burning your food to a tasteless crisp, enrol in a cookery class, learn from a loved one, watch some cooking channels and also get familiar with YouTube for a wealth of inspiration and tutorial videos. Keep trying. You can do it and your health and family will thank you for it!

- Wise up as to what you are buying in the supermarket. Read the ingredients on EVERYTHING. If the ingredient list is long and full of chemicals, additives, preservatives, synthetics, emulsifiers, flavour enhancers, mould prohibitors and words that you cannot pronounce, it is best to completely avoid that particular product. The ideal ingredients list should have a handful of natural ingredients, no additives etc. and should be easily comprehended.

- Avoid boiling and frying your food and opt instead for steaming, grilling or baking.
- Store your food in glass containers. Avoid plastic!
- Make small changes:

✓ Switch the table salt to pink Himalayan salt and the white sugar to coconut sugar or date sugar.

✓ Avoid sugar-free, no added sugar or sugar substitutes.

✓ Drink organic full fat milk or better yet plant milk instead of skimmed or fat-free dairy milk. The same goes for yoghurts etc. always choose the full-fat, plain and plant-based versions when possible. You can always top with or add in fresh fruit etc. at home.

✓ Avoid gum, candy, foods and drink containing aspartame or acesulfame K. The evidence is strong on how dangerous these chemicals are to our systems.

- Buy products in glass containers as opposed to plastic. If plastic is the only option, ensure it is BPA free.
- Drink water (and where possible pure, organic squash, raw/plant milk, fresh juice) from glass bottles.

- Find out the PH levels of the water that you drink. A PH level from 7 and above entails that the water is alkaline and healthier to consume. If you can get a water filter that mineralises and alkalises your water, that is even better. A reverse osmosis water filters is a great start.

- Get authentic raw, unheated, unpasteurised, cold extracted, organic, Fairtrade and GMO-free honey. This way you can ensure you are getting honey that is full of all the minerals, vitamins and enzymes it naturally contains as opposed to nutrient void, sweet slop.

- Always purchase Fair Trade and organic where possible.

- If you are a meat eater (this includes fish), know where your meat is coming from. I am a big supporter of local farms that have pasture-raised animals fed on organic produce. Here you can see how they are raised, question what they eat and be informed as to how humanely they are slaughtered. The meat we eat should have led as happy, healthy and as natural a life as possible. The animals should also be slaughtered in as humanely, stress-free and painlessly a manner as possible. Remember we are what we eat and we absorb the energy of what we eat. Keep meat consumption minimal, make sure it is wild/organic and from local farms that genuinely respect the lives of the animals.

- Forget the diet, eat sensibly and enjoy your food. The easiest way to go about this is starting with foods that are not packaged. Fruits and vegetables should make up the bulk of your diet. Following from this ensure you include: organic herbs, grass-fed butter, raw cheese, raw milk/plant milk, organic cold pressed extra virgin oils (olive, coconut, avocado, hemp), high quality pre and probiotics, healthy grains (amaranth, spelt, quinoa, wild rice, buckwheat, teff), fermented foods (kimchi, kefir, sauerkraut, tempeh, miso), nuts and seeds. Aim to avoid excess wine, sugar, salt, coffee, sodas etc.

- If you are not hungry, simply do not eat. You do not need to eat because 'time' indicates that you must. Listen to your body and nourish it when and only when it is hungry.

- Replace your microwave with a steamer or a toaster oven. In addition, having a slow cooker with an adjustable temperature setting is a quick, healthy and super easy way to make some seriously delicious dishes.

- Allow a day or so for light eating where you replace one or two meals with water or water and lemon/lime. This allows the internal organs a little reprieve and a chance to reset. Once you are accustomed to doing this add in 1-2 days of fasting over a period of 12-16 hours per week. The science on the health benefits of intermittent fasting show the numerous advantages of making intermittent fasting a part of your life.

- Try to get some sun each day. It is good for the soul AND it is the best form of Vitamin D. Anything from 20 minutes upwards on exposed skin is a great start.

- Invest in high quality, whole food based nutritional supplements. Do your research properly before making any decisions. You can always call the companies to enquire about how the products are made, how they should be used and most importantly, what's in them.

- Take some time each day to tune into your body. Nourish it with what it responds well to and eliminate what it does not like.

- Rest! We are a society that over does everything from food to lifestyle. This is why it is sometimes so hard to wind down. Plan a day where you can stay home once a week, lounge around, nap, and do nothing except replenish yourself.

Spirituality: As a Christian, I believe in God and all of His wondrous works. When life is at its most challenging, it is to Him that I run to for guidance, for comfort, for strength and for reassurance.

We all have different ways of communicating with God. When in constant communication with Him, I believe that we offset a lot of unnecessary pain IF we listen to His voice and follow His guidance.

Sometimes all we need to do is to listen to His message, read His word or be blessed in His presence through song. God is here and He loves us. There is nothing more cleansing and freeing than being in His presence. If you are a person who benefits from fellowship with other believers, seek to find a good bible believing church, with members and a Pastor with an active and genuine passion for God. Look for a Pastor who has a love of people and a greater love of God. Be prayerful about the choice of church you are seeking. You will know if it is the Spirit of God is active a church when you are humbled, drawn close to God and feel the constant desire to be at one with Him through song, prayer and praise and worship. The Pastor should preach the word of God in Spirit and in Truth, the way it was intended, focusing only on pleasing God and urging us as Gods people to be more Christ like. It would be a benefit if the church has a mid-week teaching service such as a bible study and a prayer session where you can learn and grow in Christ through the word of God, in a loving, judgement free environment.

When you do feel led to join a Church, pray about what God wants you to do for Him and how He wants you to do it. Then, enjoy being in the House of the Lord. It is a wonderful place to be.

If Church is not the way in which you seek to commune with God, simply spending time with Him each day in solitude and in meditation, talking to Him, acknowledging Him, following

His lead and His will in all that you do is enough. Seek to live a good and spiritual life through following His commandments and you will be blessed.

Fit: Exercise can be very hard to commit to in our daily lives IF we overcomplicate it. Simply put, if we try to keep ourselves physically moving as much as we can in the day we are halfway there.

> ➢ Walk as much as possible. Play with the children. Run with the dogs, with a friend or on your own. Join that class you have been wanting to try. Sign up for that fitness challenge. Go to that dance group you've been dreaming of joining or learn that sport! Start walking and hiking across beautiful spots in the country. Find something you love to do and just keep moving.
>
> ➢ Exercise should not be a chore. If it is, you have got to figure out how to change that so that you can equate moving your body to feelings of happiness, strength and relaxation.
>
> ➢ Get a fitness journal and start by writing down your health and fitness goals. Be clear, specific and include a deadline by which you will accomplish your goals. In this journal, take a note of how much activity you

do each day, from walking to work, cleaning the house or doing a training session in the gym. Everything counts. From here you can assess how much you are doing and make the necessary changes to attain your goal. Aim to make notes for 7-14 days to properly analyse your behavioural patterns and make changes where needed. Remember you should be aiming for one hour daily of moderate to intense exercise!

➢ Do not get into the habit of weighing yourself. It is pointless as there are so factors upon which our weight can fluctuate daily (hydration being one) and if these principles are not understood one can become quickly demotivated if the scale is not moving in the desired direction even though progress is being made. Instead observe the positive changes your body has to exercise by the way your clothes fit, how you look in pictures and how you feel. If you work better with numbers get a proper body fat assessment completed by a professional health care provider/personal trainer or simply grab the measuring tape and take your own measurements starting around your waist. Aim to do these measurements on the same points every 4-6 weeks.

➤ If you are eating well, with the addition of a great exercise regimen, good sleep and proper stress management, you are well on your way to attaining a fantastic body that looks great, is strong and can easily ward off disease.

➤ Aim to be active most days of the week and at least one day of the week you should allow your body to rest. Start with thirty minutes daily. You should work up a little sweat and after should experience a flush of those feel good happy endorphin hormones! If you do not see results immediately that is because good things take time. Allow yourself three months as a minimum to start seeing changes. When you do see the changes, even if they are small to start with, continue on and do not stop until you reach your goals!

➤ Mix up your training and give yourself at least one day off in the week to rest completely. Your fitness and physical activity regimen should include a blend of flexibility (stretching), aerobic (running, walking, swimming) and anaerobic (weight lifting, sprinting) exercises in order to get a good functional training regimen in place. Aim for 60 minutes of moderate to intense exercise each day.

> Research your body type. Google is great for this! Aim to adhere to the suggestions of the exercises best suited to your body type.

> Stay active and have fun doing it! Always get the children involved where possible. A healthy and fit family is a happy family.

Action: Try something new, and if you can do this daily, that is even better. Imagine how awesome life would be if each day we consciously made the effort to open up ourselves to trying new things! Simply start by saying yes more often and allowing yourself to try new things without too much reservation. Variety is truly the spice of life.

It is always good to grow, to learn, to discover and to stretch ourselves into new dimensions. Start with making an 'Action List'. Write down everything you want to experience during your time here on planet earth. It could be as simple as reading a book on a lovely, sunny summer's day whilst laying down on freshly cut grass, to exploring caves in an exotic far away land, or swimming in the sea with wild dolphins. Write and do not stop until your action list fills you with excitement and that buzz that calls you to action. Put it somewhere that you can see daily and make sure that you have written it beautifully. It should inspire you to do something new each day.

By simply doing this you are calling your desires into being.

The benefits to answering your inner call to action are endless and the rewards we reap immediately and also later on down the line are positively immense! Now you have some tips to get you started on this wonderful journey. I wish you every success!

Day 1

Happy: Appreciation opens the door to a multitude of blessings. Take a walk in the sunshine. Allow the sun to soak into your skin. Feel its warmth. Inhale the fresh air. Allow yourself to breathe, fully and deeply. Listen to the beauty in the bird song. Give thanks for life and the wonders it brings. Acknowledge the magnificence it bestows in the wondrous nature around you and the simple way in which it refreshes your soul. There is always something that we can appreciate and when we take the time to give appreciation for even the smallest things, we are given more to be appreciative about. Isn't that wonderful! Daily on waking and before falling into a peaceful rest, find a few things to appreciate. In this simple acknowledgement you will come to appreciate the fact that life, in all of its complexity, is truly good.

Bible Verse: 1 Thessalonians 5:18- In everything give thanks; for this is God's will for you in Christ Jesus.

Healthy: Adzuki beans encompass a powerful nutritious blend and benefit several health conditions such as diabetes, diarrhoea, high blood cholesterol and fluid retention. To prepare adzuki beans, soak them in a glass bowl of filtered water with the juice of a fresh lemon (one cup of water to one teaspoon of lemon juice) for at least 24 hours, changing the water a minimum of one time in the process. You can also use apple cider vinegar or pink Himalayan salt instead of lemon juice.

Soaking the beans helps to get rid of phytic acid, indigestible sugars which can cause gas, and tannins. It also assists in removing the anti-nutrient barrier in the bean and allows you to easily absorb and digest the nutrients in your food.

You can sprout adzuki beans by placing fresh beans in a spouting jar or container and watering them with fresh, filtered and/boiled water each day. After a few days you will start to see a little sprout (tail) and after a day or so more, little leaves. These nutrient rich sprouts are bursting with vitamins and minerals and are delicious as a stand-alone snack or with a lemon juice and olive oil dressing.

Adzuki beans are delicious in soups, salads, and steamed vegetables or eaten as an accompaniment to rice, pasta, meat, fish or polenta.

Fit: Aerobic activity such as walking, running, cycling or swimming are the most simple and common ways to keep fit and feel great. Go for a scenic walk in nature for 30 minutes. Don't plan the route in full. Allow some room for exploration. Don' set a pace. Permit your body to lead you as fast or as slowly as it wants too. Feel your feet as you trod on the earth. Swing your arms gently. Breathe deeply, allowing your stomach muscles to expand and relax. Stand proudly and walk tall. Most importantly allow your body to relax into this gentle and revitalizing form of physical activity, as you profit both mentally and physically from your walk. Do this as often as you like and at least once a week.

Action: Create a piece of art that inspires you. Paint, cut, stick, mold and do whatever gets your creative juices flowing. Decorate your master piece in a beautiful frame. Place this inspirational piece of art somewhere that you can see it daily in your home or place of work.

It should make you smile. It should uplift and inspire you and most importantly it should encourage you to strive towards greatness in all areas of your life. Remember you are awesome. Let the encompassment of your greatness reflect in this piece.

Day 2

Happy: Believing you are worthy of everything good and great and wonderful is the start of an amazing journey. Create a mood board. On this board, you will place only pictures, inspirational quotes and words that make you feel happy and joyous. You can get these pictures, quotes, and words from online, magazines, leaflets or you can draw them up yourself. Get creative. Make it a beautiful board. Look at it every day and imagine the things you have placed on it in real time. Watch as your dreams become your reality. Believe in yourself. You were born destined for greatness.

Bible Verse: Mark 11:24- Therefore I tell you, whatever you ask for in prayer, believe that you have received it, and it will be yours.

Healthy: Buckwheat is a delicious, gluten-free grain that is truly amazing with a dash of seasoning and a hearty dollop of grass-fed butter melted over it. It is a great substitute for rice, pasta, or potatoes.

Buckwheat is a nutrient dense grain that helps to lower blood glucose and cholesterol levels. It has high levels of tryptophan which helps to promote a good night's sleep. Before cooking, soak for 24 hours in a glass bowl of filtered and/or boiled water using one cup of water to one teaspoon of freshly squeezed lemon juice. This will help to break down the anti-nutrients and hard to digest components of the buckwheat whilst simultaneously releasing the highly beneficial nutrients. Buckwheat flakes make a delicious breakfast as an equally healthy alternative to oats.

Fit: Body weight training is a simple, free and effective way to get and stay in shape. Your body mass is sufficient enough to give you the extra weight you need for a great strength training session. Push ups, planks, sit-ups, tricep dips, squats, lunges, tuck jumps, jumping jacks, burpees or high knees are just some of the exercises that you can do in a body weight session. YouTube will become a great resource as you watch videos of what sort of exercises you can do no matter what your fitness level. Aim to do at least three bodyweight exercises (to failure: meaning that you stop only when you are physically unable to do another repetition with the proper form) in every training session.

Action: What is the one thing that you can do to make yourself absolutely BEAUTIFUL from the inside out? Sleep more? Eat better? Let go of unhealthy thoughts? Stress a bit less? Laugh a lot more? Accept yourself exactly as you are right now? See the best in everyone and in everything? Be more gratuitous? Today commit to yourself to do just that one thing that will make you beautiful from the inside out!

Day 3

Happy: We should all strive towards carefree, tranquil and gratifying living. Nowadays we are so well trained to be on the go 24/7 that when we find ourselves with spare time, we find it difficult to relax, and in some cases, we cannot. This is partly attributable to why our stress levels are high and we sometimes feel out of control. We literally need to learn to let go and to be okay with not controlling every hour of the day. When we fill each hour of the day with activity, we allow little to no time for rest and rejuvenation. You will note that when you are well rested how much better your day flows, how calm and happy you are and how you are able to make sound decisions from a place of peace.

Plan to have a *guilt free* lie in for at least a couple of hours at some point this week. Do absolutely nothing. Lounge about as though you have not a care in the world. It is great for the soul! Start the day with a hot shower and fresh clean clothes. Put on some gentle music or read an uplifting book. Light a candle or burn some incense (either option should be chemical free). Indulge in the art of nothingness. Snooze if you desire to. Wrap yourself in a warm, soft blanket and forget about your worries. Enjoy something wholesome and decadent to eat. Be in perfect peace. Allow yourself at least one day each week to de-stress, and do absolutely nothing. It is rejuvenating, refreshing and vital to not only your physical and mental health but it is food for your soul.

Bible Verse: 1 Peter 5:7- Casting all your care upon him; for He careth for you.

Healthy: Oral health plays a vital role in the overall well-being of our body. Coconut oil is a great addition to your oral care routine. Oil pulling is an ancient remedy that uses natural substances to clean and detoxify your teeth and gums. Coconut oil pulling can help to whiten teeth naturally. It is beneficial in improving gums and removing harmful bacteria by binding to plaque on the teeth some of which lead to tooth decay and gum disease. Oil pulling can also help to prevent erosion of the enamel after bouts of vomiting. Simply rinse your mouth, and gargle with coconut oil after each episode of vomiting to protect the enamel of the teeth. Oil pulling is super easy. Using a food grade raw, organic, cold-pressed, virgin coconut oil simply swish a teaspoon of oil in your mouth for up to 20 minutes. Spit and rinse with cool water or follow up with a brush of Himalayan pink salt for that extra clean. Never swallow the coconut oil that you have gargled with as it full of toxins.

Fit: Cycling is a great individual, team or family physical activity to undertake. Most cities now have a 'Rent a Bicycle' scheme where you can rent a bicycle for a set price or even free. Don't have a car? Why not invest in a quality bicycle? If you have children you can get a bicycle seat for them which attaches to the front or back of the bicycle, or a bicycle trailer until they can ride along with you. Some employers offer 'Cycle to Work' schemes which can assist towards the cost of a cycle.

Further, many local councils offer cycle training courses to help you learn how to cycle safely and confidently on the road. There are also spin classes held at gyms or leisure centres which are a great option for staying fit. Cycling is a great calorie burner. It is low impact, can be done with the entire family, and is an environmentally friendly form of transport.

The best thing about cycling aside from the fact that you are getting an amazing workout is the fact that you can cycle for miles and miles exploring beautiful places, embarking on adventure after adventure, whilst keeping fit.

Action: Confidence can take us from a position of fear to a position of authority. Give yourself permission to be bold and more confident in your day to day activities and interactions with others. It is simply a matter of practice, one of familiarity. If we become accustomed to doing something, our confidence grows. By exposing yourself to experiences that can specifically help to build your confidence you will slowly but surely begin to transform for the better in that area.

Think of situations in which you are less confident and self-assured. Step out of your comfort zone by allowing yourself to engage in such situations more frequently in order to build your confidence. For example, you may not be a confident public speaker. Joining a public speaking group is a great way of building you confidence in this area. You will note that after a few attempts you are not so nervous or dubious of your ability to speak publicly, and may even enjoy it more than anticipated.

Take note of your increased self-esteem and your improved sense of self. This newfound status of confidence will see you doing things you were previously hesitant to do and living a life full of varied experiences and delightful challenges. Today, think of an area where you lack confidence. What is one thing you can do to help increase your confidence in this area? Now, do that one thing!

Day 4

Happy: Detox your mind! Free yourself from bitterness, anger, jealousy and strife. If there are broken relationships in your life either fix them or let them go. Keep in your realm only those who love you, lift you up, inspire you, motivate you and bring out the very best in you. Be around happy, loving people. You are worth this!

Bible Verse: Philippians 4:8- Finally, brethren, whatsoever things are true, whatsoever things are honest, whatsoever things are just, whatsoever things are pure, whatsoever things are lovely, whatsoever things are of good report; if there be any virtue, and if there be any praise, think on these things.

Healthy: Detox! Try it for a week. See how absolutely amazing you feel after. Every part of you will feel restored, revived and renewed. Eliminate from your diet and environment the following:

1. Useless background noise.

2. Negative and depressing news from radio, TV, magazines etc.

3. Social media.

4. Sleeping with the TV, phone, computer, radio, watch or any electronic devices on or near you. Keep them off or in another room. Many people are becoming clued up about the dangers of electronic magnetic fields (EMF's). It's best to keep your exposure reduced as much as possible.

5. Do away with smoking and alcohol.

6. Try to clean without using chemicals make your own cleaning sprays from essential oils, vinegar or baking soda.

7. Cut out swearing and profanity from your language. Avoid programmes and people who swear excessively, engage in negative self-talk and gossip. If you have nothing nice to say, nothing that builds you up or lifts up another, then remain in peaceful silence.

8. Ban Junk food! Read the ingredients on the packages of the food you are purchasing. Become familiar with what you are putting in your body. No junk this week!

9. Cleanse internally with a no meat, bread or sugar diet. Similar to a Daniel Fast in the Bible. Alternatively, you

can choose to also include a green smoothie or fruit and vegetable juice each day to your meal plan.

10. Replace every negative thought with a positive thought!

11. Book time in your schedule for at least thirty minutes of rest and relaxation daily. Do something that will make you laugh every day.

12. Shed the weight and toxicity of emotional burdens. You know what works best for you. For some it is journaling, for some it is having a good hearty cry, for others it is just coming to terms with certain things, acknowledging them and being at peace with letting go. Find what works for you and do it.

Fit: Discover somewhere new! Get your running shoes out and go for a run around the block. Explore the town or city that you live in. Pick the pace up a bit. Feel your heart pumping and enjoy the feel of your skin sweating, cleansing you of toxins and keeping you cool whilst you enjoy a bit of exploration. You can do the same on your bicycle.

Feeling for a bit of adventure? Why not explore your surroundings on a boat? The summer time is a great time to do this. Being out on the water is refreshing and calming. Get in a paddleboat or canoe and start your discovery! Always carry some water with you, wear a high visibility shirt/life jacket and be aware of your surroundings! Most importantly live in the moment! You're expanding your horizons and doing something wonderful.

Action: Decide to appreciate yourself. You are marvellous! Engage in the art of self-care. From today going forward, always make sure you are well groomed, well dressed and well nourished. Think about all the things you love and appreciate the most about yourself. Every morning, take some time to gaze in the mirror, smile and simply appreciate yourself just as you are. Do this often. It feels just as good, if not a tad bit better when you recognise and own your amazingness.

Day 5

Happy: Essential oils are used in aromatherapy as a means of using natural scents for treating a variety of ailments. Some great essential oils to have in your home are clary sage, lemongrass, peppermint, lavender, frankincense, eucalyptus, chamomile, tea tree, and geranium. You can always pop into a local health food store to try sampling some of the essential oil scents before committing to a purchase. Learn which ones work for you, uplift and refresh you. To enjoy, simply follow the instructions on each essential oil bottle before use. Dilute a few drops of your chosen essential oil with carrier oil (like sweet almond oil, grapeseed oil or jojoba oil) and rub into your skin for an instantaneous happy hit!

Bible Verse: Deuteronomy 7:9- Know therefore that the LORD your God, He is God, the faithful God, who keeps His covenant and His lovingkindness to a thousandth generations with those who love Him and keep His commandments.

Healthy: Emotions! How are you feeling right now? Is there anything that you can do to change how you feel to feel even better? How does your body feel right now? Are you tensed or relaxed? Take a deep breath and allow your muscles to fully relax in each and every part of your body, from your scalp, forehead, cheeks and right down to your toes, completely relax. Do an emotion check by simply by assessing the state of your body and where you note there is tension, try to relax and let go.

Eat well for your emotions by also paying attention to emotional eating. Make a note of whether you overeat or under eat during periods of stress and make an effort to maintain healthy eating habits even when the going gets tough.

Think of ways that you can replace eating with movement or something that will deter you from eating based on the emotional need to do so and do this when the need to eat because of emotional stresses arise.

Fit: Try a different form of exercise from the list below. It should be an activity you have not done before.

Cross fit	TRX	Plyo	Barre
Powerlifting	Team sports	P 90 x	Tae Bo
Fight Klub	Dance	Tai Chi	Hot Pod Yoga
Insanity	Bounce Fit	Boot camp	Nordic walking
Pilates	Wild Swimming		Rock Climbing
Cycling	Spin	Boxing	Kickboxing
Aquarobics	Fencing	Diving	Trampolining
Gymnastics	Rowing		

Action: Entertain some friends or family this month. Decide on a day, a time, a menu and a theme. Enjoy the feeling of giving back and providing joy for others. Make a real effort to see to it that your guests are well fed, properly entertained and luxuriously pampered. Enjoy the little things in life, like giving with love and joy and from a pure heart and expecting nothing back.

Day 6

Happy: What is it that you fear the most? What is the one thing that you give are subconsciously giving permission to inadvertently control your life? We often times allow fear to control us, to a point where it becomes a debilitating master. We are the rulers of our destiny and the conquerors over all. Fear has no place in our greatness. Seek to root it out and allow yourself to shine. Seek out what you fear and conquer it and then your fear shall be no more.

Bible Verse: 2 Timothy 1:7- For God hath not given us the spirit of fear, but of power, and of love, and of a sound mind.

Healthy: Fermented vegetables such as kimchi and sauerkraut are full of healthy probiotics which are great for our gut health and contributes to increased immunity. Fermented foods are full of microflora (healthy bacteria), are extremely cost effective as they are cheaper and, in some cases, more powerful than store bought probiotics. They can also gently detoxify the body and as such can lead to weight loss. Not to mention the fact that they taste amazing.

Some delicious fermented foods like kefir, tempeh or kimchi can be easily added to your diet and can be made at home in very little time and with minimal effort. A few fermented foods to try are: kefir, kombucha, natto, tempeh, yogurt, pickles, sauerkraut, miso and yogurt.

Fit: Find a friend who you know has not exercised in a long time and needs the extra support to start. Be that support system. Go for regular walks, swims, dancing or whatever it takes to get your friend up and moving to become fit and healthy.

The most important thing is to ensure that you are both having fun as this will ensure longevity and continuity! Align your goals and commit to accomplishing them together. Make a commitment and see it through for both yourself and your friend until you are both fighting fit!

Action: Choose to forget the hurt, the pain and the things that bring you down. Acknowledge the pain and then let it go. Focus on your happy; whatever makes you beam with joy from deep within. Fixate your mind only on what will bring you abundant joy and peace. Choose to be happy, choose to be at peace, and choose to focus on feeling good. Your focus on happiness will only bring you more things to be happy about. In and of itself, that is reason enough to start being joyful.

Day 7

Happy: The most simple and effective way to attain true happiness is to be grateful and gratuitous. Give thanks for what you have, for what you have had and for what is on the way! As you are blessed with each new day, thank your way through it. Whatever good comes your way, whatever you are fortunate to have or to experience, for all the joy you have and for all that you will be give thanks now. The happy feelings should arise immediately.

Bible Verse: Romans 8:28 - And we know that all things work together for good to them that love God, to them who are the called according to his purpose.

Healthy: Go green. Green beverages are amazing at alkalizing the body and providing a host of numerous health benefits. Green beverages provide you with a vast array of vitamins and minerals in addition to the added benefits of probiotics and prebiotics. Green powders are nutritional powerhouses. There are also fermented powders that contain prebiotics which nourish the probiotics, antioxidants and digestive enzymes. Look for alfalfa, barley, spirulina, wheatgrass, chlorella, hemp protein powder, alfalfa powder, and spinach to name a few. They should always be GMO-Free and organic. You can make your own green drinks by juicing celery, cucumbers, spinach, kale, lemons, broccoli, green apples, pears, or green peppers, wheatgrass etc. and blending in avocadoes and melons.

Fit: Grounding workouts are so beautifully refreshing. Once you have tried a grounding workout you will regularly integrate it into part of your routine. Grounding is also known as Earthing, and it basically entails walking barefoot on the earth, sand, soil, grass etc. When grounding, there is a feeling of being at one with and totally connected to the earth. There are numerous health benefits to be obtained from grounding such as a reduction in chronic pain and relieving of muscle tension. Grounding is perfect for the active person. In a clean area, free from debris, try doing a simple bodyweight or stretching workout (yoga or even yoga-lates) barefoot on grass or damp soil. Try grounding first thing in the morning on the freshly damp morning dew.

Action: Gratitude lists are an amazing tool in helping us to be cognizant of just how much we really have. In a journal, notebook or even on your phone, just before you go to bed or as you start the day, jot down as many things as you can think of that you are grateful for. It will soon be easy to see just how truly rich you really are as you start and end your day on a gratuitous note!

Day 8

Happy: You can heal your wounds. The ones that we bury so deep inside of us we often forget that they are there. The ones that will take a considerable amount of effort to deal with but the ones that will also offer us the most freedom and joy once healed. Now is the time to start. We all carry pain, hurt and regret of the past from things that we have done and things that others have done to us. What we should endeavour to avoid is allowing the negative memories of these experiences to reside within us. Aside from choosing to forgive, counselling or journaling your way through some of your most difficult experiences, decide that you will not allow them to bring you down emotionally. One proactive and positive way to use the bad for good is to identify how these negative scenarios have made you stronger, braver, more independent and more aware of yourself. Is there any good that has come out of what you have been through? Is there a way you can help someone else because of what you have been through? Can you colour the bad good and come away stronger, more resilient and happier? Heal your wounds by deciding that you will use all the challenges you have overcome for your betterment and choose to forge forward to a better present.

Bible Verse: Hebrews 13:5-6- Let your conduct be without covetousness; be content with such things as you have. For He Himself has said, 'I will never leave you nor forsake you.' So, we may boldly say: 'The LORD is my helper; I will not fear. What can man do to me?'

Healthy: Hemp seeds are delicious, soft and mildly flavoured seeds packed full of nutrition. They are rich in healthy fats, protein, and various minerals. Hemp seeds are a great protein source, as more than 25% of their total calories are protein. Hemp seeds help to reduce the risk of heart disease and can benefit skin conditions such as dry skin, eczema, and itchiness.

Hemp seeds are considered to be a complete protein source because they contain all the essential amino acids, which is rare in the plant kingdom. This is important as essential amino acids are not produced in the body and need to be obtained from the diet.

Enjoy hemp seeds on their own, in flapjacks, blended into a smoothie, blended to make your own hemp milk, or sprinkled on top of porridge or yoghurt.

Fit: High-intensity interval training is a training technique in which you give all-out, one hundred percent effort through quick, intense bursts of exercise, followed by short, and sometimes active recovery periods. This type of training gets and keeps your heart rate up and burns more fat in less time as opposed to cardiovascular activity. The great thing about HIIT is that you can basically HIIT in any format. From swimming, cycling, circuits to running you can HIIT anywhere such as the gym, the park, from home or your office with little to no equipment! If you are pressed for time, it is the most efficient workout muscle toning out and fat loss.

Action: Get a health check. Find out what your bone density, body fat, body muscle percentage, blood cholesterol, blood pressure, blood sugar levels, resting heart rate readings, allergens, blood type and hormone levels are.

If you are within the normal parameter's keep up the good work. If not, well done for taking the first step on our journey to becoming healthier, happier and fitter by finding out where you are, now all you need to do is to start to implement healthy lifestyle choices.

Following functional medicine, and implementing therapies such as nutritional therapy, homeopathy and aromatherapy in addition to focusing on emotional healing is a great place to start improving your health holistically.

Day 9

Happy: Intelligence requires that we commit ourselves to the continuous art of learning in various capacities and differing dimensions. Challenge your mind today. Learn something new. Select a new hobby that is interesting, difficult and stimulating. Even if it may seem a bit perplexing, initially, you will profit from exercising your brain, improving your memory and enhancing your overall mental well-being and later on down the line potentially offsetting dementia.

Bible Verse: Lamentations 3:22-23- Because of the Lord's great love we are not consumed, for his compassions never fail. They are new every morning; great is your faithfulness.

Healthy: Incan berries also known as gooseberries are crammed full of vitamins C and A, iron, niacin, and phosphorous. For a berry, Incan berries are high in protein and fibre. They provide antioxidant effects, defend against cancer, counter bacteria, have a protective effect on the kidneys and liver, can lower fever and blood sugar levels, help to modulate immune function, reduce inflammation and may have weight loss benefits.

Astounding for one little berry! You can find dried Incan berries in most health food stores which are delicious in a homemade fruit and nut mix.

Fit: Interval training is a type of physical training that involves a series of low intensity to high-intensity exercises interspersed with brief periods of rest. The high-intensity periods are typically anaerobic exercises (think sprints), while the recovery periods involve lower intensity activity (like walking or jogging). You can do a simple interval training workout at a park, pool, on the track or on the bike.

Example: Sprint for 30 seconds, then jog or walk for 10 seconds. Repeat 5 times. Rest for 5 minutes and then start again. Do three full sets. Be sure to cool down and enjoy a nice, long full body stretch after.

Action: Interview yourself. Sit down over a cup of tea and ponder upon those deep questions about yourself, such as your beliefs, your friends, the choices you've made and if you are the best person you can possibly be. Ask probing questions and give honest answers. You will soon discover some amazing things and will have the ability to make the changes you need to improve your life and current circumstances. Don't rush this time with yourself. At the end of this session you should come away knowing yourself better. In the process make a plan of action as to how you will ensure you make the best of life going forward. Make your story good to tell and great to hear!

Day 10

Happy: Joy is a state of being that we should endeavour to encompass at all times. We can find joy in the simple things, the sun shining, the smell of freshly cut grass or freshly roasted coffee, indulging in a good book, cuddles from a loved one, laughing with your children, watching an inspiring movie, or eating your favourite foods. We should seek to enjoy and to spread joy each and every day. In all things we should be joyful. When we radiate joy, we spread it unconsciously to those around us and to those who need it. Smile at the lonesome elderly person sitting alone, pay for something for someone who looks like they could use the help, buy a meal or some clothing for a homeless person, donate some time in the animal shelter, sit and talk to someone who could use an ear, give without expecting anything back. On the path to becoming more joyful, we elevate those who we meet along the way and that is a beautiful thing.

Bible Verse: Romans 15:13- May the God of hope fill you with all joy and peace as you trust in Him so that you may overflow with Hope by the power of the Holy Spirit.

Healthy: 100% fruit juice is full of essential vitamins and minerals. Both "from concentrate" and "not from concentrate" juices are pasteurised to remove probable pathogens that may have been in the fruit. The pasteurisation process involves rapidly heating the juice to kill any pathogens but can also deplete the juice of vitamins and minerals.

"Not from concentrate" juice is made by juicing the fruit and then pasteurising it. "From concentrate" juice is made from juicing the fruit and then filtering it through a processor that extracts the water. When the juice is ready to be packaged and sold, water is added back into the concentrated juice and it is then pasteurised.

If you are going to drink commercial juice, avoid *juice drinks* and juices with added flavourings, sugars or sweeteners, which are often present in mixed juice drink blends. Simply read the ingredients list and look for juice concentrates that say they are 100 percent juice on the label. Organic, cold pressed juices are a great choice if you cannot juice your own fruits and vegetables. Half a cup of juice is equal to one serving of fruit and vegetables.

Fit: Implement this workout into your training regimen this week and see how great you feel afterwards!

<u>**Full body Workout:**</u>

Complete three rounds!

- o   1 minute of jump rope
- o   30 seconds of jump squats
- o   30 seconds plank
- o   2 minutes of fast jogging/cycling (in place or on the treadmill/watt or spin bike)
- o   30 seconds of jumping jacks
- o   30 seconds of alternating lunges
- o   30 seconds of push ups
- o   30 seconds of Russian Twists

To make the workout more challenging, adjust the incline to a challenging height on a treadmill or add ankle weights and hand weights. When you do this workout remember you are going for it with 100% effort, so in each set take no breaks until after you have completed the set, keep going and give it your absolute all. It is a great conditioning, cardiovascular and mental workout! Well done.

Action: Journaling is an unquestionably remarkable form of free therapy. You can jot a phrase, a paragraph or pour out your soul onto numerous pages of internal verbiage. Just get it out. Hold nothing back. Allow yourself to be authentic with how certain emotions surface. Don't be a hero. Cry, shout, and laugh as the needs presents. Feel how free you feel after, mentally and emotionally. When you practice journaling regularly, you will gain more clarity and insight as you will be able to rationalise things better when you get it down on paper. Try journaling first thing in the morning or just before you go to bed at night to start and end your day with a clear mind. At the end of each journaling session you can, if you decide to, rip up the pages of what you have just written and in doing that let it stand as a symbol of release.

Day 11

Happy: Keep a memory box with all your favourite things inside. Don't have a collection? Make one! Get beautiful things, things that smell gorgeous, things that are lovely to touch, things that make you smile, things that you adore and things that you can pass down to your children, or that have been passed onto you. Fill it with anything and everything that brings you a feeling of love, joy, happiness, and calm. This memory box should be one that is a delight to open and one that warms your heart, brings a smile to your face, and gratitude to your heart.

Bible Verse: Ephesians 4:26- Be ye angry, and sin not: let not the sun go down upon your wrath.

Healthy: Kombucha is known as the "Immortal Health Elixir" by the Chinese. It originated in the Far East around 2,000 years ago. Kombucha is a fermented beverage of black tea and sugar with tremendous health benefits. This solution of sugar and tea is fermented by a bacteria and yeast commonly known as the "SCOBY" (a symbiotic colony of bacteria and yeast).

After fermentation, kombucha becomes carbonated and contains vinegar, b-vitamins, enzymes, probiotics and a high concentration of acid (acetic, gluconic and lactic), which are linked with the following benefits: improved digestion, weight loss, increased energy, cleansing and detoxification, immune support, reduced joint pain and cancer prevention. You can make kombucha yourself at home or buy it at most health food stores. Kombucha can be quite strong so start off with half a cup or so a day.

Fit: Kickboxing is a group of stand-up combat sports primarily based on kicking and punching. Traditionally it was developed from Karate, Muay Thai, Khmer Boxing, and Western boxing.

In addition to being practised as a contact sport or for self-defense, kickboxing is also a great form of whole-body fitness. Many gyms offer kickboxing, combat, boxercise and various forms of martial arts keep fit classes guaranteed to make you break a sweat and shed some pounds.

Action: A random act of kindness towards others is another way of being kind to yourself. What goes around comes around! Choose three people and commit to a random act of kindness for each. Gift them with something that you know they either need or want. Make sure it is something wonderful. Genuinely enjoy the process of thinking about what they would love, purchasing, making it or doing it for them and then surprising them with your wonderful gift of love. Spread kindness!

Day 12

Happy: Let it go. Let go of the pain, let go of the hurt, let go of anything and everything that brings you down. Learn to live in love. You may not know what love feels like, so teach yourself to love. Care for something, an animal, a plant, an elderly person until they thrive.

Allow yourself to be loved and to receive gratefully the love that others show and give to you. Love is kind, love is pure, it is forgiving, it is peace, it is calm and it is gentle.

Seek after the things which embrace and embody love.

Bible verse: Proverbs: 5-6- Trust in the Lord with all thine heart; and lean not unto thine own understanding. In all thy ways acknowledge him, and he shall direct thy paths.

Healthy: Use your organic lemon, orange or lime peels to make your own Vitamin C powder. Simply dry out the cleaned peels of the unwaxed fruits until they are hard. When the peels have dried, use a coffee grinder to blend them into a powder. The peels contain more Vitamin C than the actual fruit and are GMO-free if sourced accordingly. Store your Vitamin C in a glass container in the fridge.

Fit: Try your hand at long distance training. Run, swim, cycle, walk! Have a long, slow, distance training day. Run over mountains, through rivers and across fields. It's great to mix up your training programme and even better to challenge yourself to do something that you have not done before.

Make sure you are properly warmed up, nourished and hydrated before you begin your long slow distance day. Have a good stretch after and a nutrient dense and balanced meal containing some protein, fats and carbohydrates to replenish your body after all of your hard work. Aim to cycle, walk, swim or run anything upwards of three miles. There is no need to do marathon lengths unless you are actually training for one.

Action: Listen to your favourite music, dim the lights, light a candle, spray on your favourite perfume/cologne or essential oil blends, loosen up and let go of all the stress. Slowly and gently rub your temples and the side of your wrists, the palms of your hands or the bottom of your feet. Make your favourite drink and just be, just breathe and just relax. Close your eyes and smile gently. Say some positive affirmations or nothing at all. Love yourself as you are right now. Sit and revel in the sweet succulence of the present moment for as long as you can. Life is good.

Day 13

Happy: Mindfulness is becoming increasingly popular as we realise the benefits of being aware and 'present'. It allows us to centre ourselves back to a balanced state of being from which we can make the accurate choices for our current circumstances. It also highlights just how distracted we are from what is really happening in and around us. Being cognizant and mindful of how we are thinking, what we are thinking about, how we are feeling, and what we are doing at regular points throughout the day can help us to steer ourselves towards the good and positive path. Mindfulness in eating, breathing, thinking and being can be practised by just committing yourself to being aware, aware of yourself and aware of your surroundings. It is that simple.

Bible Verse: Isiah 26:3-You will keep in perfect peace those whose minds are steadfast because they trust in you.

Healthy: Trace minerals are inorganic substances, needed in small amounts to help your body function properly. Trace minerals are vital to health and provide an absolute wealth of benefits. They can increase energy levels, improve concentration, increase mental clarity, promote an increased sense of wellbeing, and promote anti-aging due to recovery nutrients. They balance, restore and rejuvenate cell life. They support a healthy thyroid gland, boost the immune system, increase circulation, cleanse, neutralise and help in liver detoxification, help oxygenate the blood and support balanced hormone levels. Trace minerals can be consumed by adding a few drops into juice or water.

Fit: Speed up your metabolism by increasing your muscle mass. Aim for workouts where you are using body weights or free weights. Push yourself until you feel like you want to stop and then do a few more repetitions. The goal here is to consistently aim to exceed your personal best. Don't always work to a set number of repetitions of each exercise (say for example, 20 jumping jacks), but listen to your body (you could probably do 50) and give yourself the chance to exceed your fitness levels and train to failure. Here is where the benefits are reaped!

If you are training in the gym and are not sure what to do ask for help. Remember you are seeking to improve yourself and there is nothing wrong (although it can be a bit daunting at times) asking for someone to show you how to use a piece of equipment (barbells, kettlebells, TRX and cable machines).

The weights area is not a men's only, young person's or hot bodies only area. It is for everyone. If this is an area in the gym that is intimidating for you, try going during the quiet times and getting familiar with the equipment and the exercises. Make an appointment with a personal trainer or fitness instructor and ask them to show you how to use the equipment properly. If there are gym floor-based classes, attend a couple during the busy and quiet times to familiarise yourself and get comfortable with being in the weights area and in the gym. This may take time but have fun in the process. Commit to adding full body weight training to your regimen three times a week. Start with 3 to 4 sets of 12-16 repetitions for each exercise, of which there should be at least 8 exercises in each weight training session. You will see, feel and bask in the glorious results of all your hard work.

Action: Massages are so great for relieving mental and physical stress and exhaustion. Better yet there are so many types of massages to choose from. Why not have a spa day, or book a few spa sessions at varying facilities and sample what's on offer? From there decide which you like best and book yourself in for a massage once or twice a month.

This part of your self-care regimen should be booked into your daily calendar and treated just as importantly as a business meeting with the CEO of your company. Take the time to see what sort of massage your body likes and from there get one monthly. If you are genuinely too busy to go out to get a massage, for a little extra more, find a masseuse who can come to you.

Day 14

Happy: Out with the old, and in with the new. Go through your home and room by room declutter and where needed redecorate. Give what you no longer need to charity. Add some lovely new pieces of clothing to your wardrobe. Choose a new look for yourself. Repaint a tired wall. Place gorgeous fresh flowers and or plants around your home to brighten and beautify it. Rearrange the furniture so that the energy flows through your home peacefully and harmoniously. Your home should be unique, attractive and gloriously serene. Change tired rugs with new ones, clean your home until it sparkles. Scent it beautifully with an essential oil diffuser. Put up paintings and pictures of good times you have had. Your home should be your haven, your 'me cave', your spot and your little piece of heaven. Take some time this week and make your home your sanctuary if you have not already done so.

Bible Verse: Job 12:7-10- But ask the animals, and they will teach you, or the birds in the sky, and they will tell you; or speak to the earth, and it will teach you, or let the fish in the sea inform you. Which of all these does not know that the hand of the LORD has done this? In His hand is the life of every creature and the breath of all mankind.

Healthy: The healthiest nuts for overall health and wellbeing are pecans, macadamia, walnuts, almonds, Brazil nuts, and pistachios. Nuts are packed with protein, fibre, essential fats and vitamins and minerals making a nutritious addition to your diet. Add them to your granola, yoghurt or enjoy as a standalone snack. Choose organic nuts in their raw plain unsalted form. You can also soak and then dehydrate your nuts and eat them in their raw state to remove harmful phytic acid and enzyme inhibitors and increase the nutritional availability.

Fit: Noting down exactly what you do when you train will give you a perfect glimpse of just how much or how little you are doing in addition to highlighting the areas that you need to focus on more. Get a notebook specifically for your gym sessions and jot down the exercise you do, repetitions, sets, intensity, any breaks you took, the length of your session etc. Further to this, focus on your nutrition as well. Jot down the snacks, drinks and meals and the quantities of each for each day. If you are a poor sleeper noting sleep patterns will also give you a clear idea how this affects your training and eating patterns. Similarly, you can do the same for stress levels! Review this diary weekly. You will be able to note patterns of your most effective and energised days. Once noted seek to replicate what you did on these days, it is a simple way to success.

Action: Nature is one of the best forms of free therapy, of self-rejuvenation, of connecting to our higher self and the higher form (God). When we convene with her, Mother Nature has a way of giving to us a peace of mind tranquillity, inner calm and bliss. From lakes to beaches, hills to meadows, forests to grasslands and woodlands there is so much that we can choose from and even more we have to be appreciative of.

Nature therapy, or spending quality uninterrupted time in nature is so rehabilitating on various levels. Choose your form and indulge frequently. Make a plan to be outside every day even when it is raining. Get some fresh air, some sun and some time in Mother Nature. You will notice how you benefit not only physically from doing so as you are keeping active, but the mental and psychological effects are positively amazing.

You never come back the same way that you have entered into nature. You are gifted sometimes with clarity, sometimes with peace, sometimes with reassurance, sometimes with the peace and quiet to hear your own inner voice advising you on something you are unsure about. The best thing is that all you really need to do is just get out there. Start today.

Day 15

Happy: To have a system of order in your life is to have organisation, sanity, clarity, routine and peace. Get your home in order; each room, each cupboard, each drawer, and each closet. Do the same for your office and your car, and even your storage units. Get your life in order, from your finances to your career and your personal relationships. Lastly but most importantly get yourself in order inclusive of your spiritual, emotional and physical states of well-being. If you need professional help from an accountant, stylist, housekeeper, life coach or counselor, then by all means employ them and make this a life changing effort to bring out the best of you!

Bible Verse: 1 Corinthians 6:19-20- Or do you not know that your body is a temple of the Holy Spirit within you, whom you have from God? You are not your own, for you were bought with a price. So, glorify God in your body.

Healthy: Olive oil is renowned for its benefits in preventing cardiovascular disease, stroke, breast cancer and heart disease, reducing high blood pressure and reducing the risk of depression and cholesterol.

To spot good brands of olive oil look for organic, cold-pressed extra virgin olive oil. Avoid plastic containers and look for organic, extra virgin olive oil in dark green glass containers or in packaging that shields it from light.

Olive oil is best used sprinkled over salads, in dressings or as a dip for bread. Ideally, it should not be heated or used to cook with.

Fit: Aim to really define your external oblique abdominal muscles and add further definition to your abdominals. Evaluate your training routine and turn one session into an obstacle course. Try standing side bends, moving sideways around objects on your hands without using your legs, pulling yourself up a rope, jumping side to side over a bar or plyometric box and then sprinting, going from side planks into push ups, rolling from side to side and then exploding into a jump! Make it fun and make it so that you are really targeting these core abdominal muscles on a frequent basis weekly.

Action: Organise a fun day out for yourself and a couple of your closest family or friends. Go somewhere different, somewhere that you have always yearned to visit. Create memories. Plan everything in advance from the transport to food, and even sleeping accommodation if needed. Plan what you will wear and make sure to look and feel amazing on this day. When this day comes, milk every minute of it and ensure that you have a glorious time no matter what. Take pictures to add to your mood board. Enjoy life and thoroughly enjoy the day!

Day 16

Happy: Peace and prayer go hand in hand. When you pray, you gain peace. When you are in peace you seek to be constantly prayerful because you know that you are in union with God. It is a great idea to have a quiet and serene place in your home, just for yourself. Dedicate a corner of a room, or even an entire room that will allow you to be at one with yourself and with God. In this spot meditate on the words of God. Be still. Just be. Enjoy the calm that comes with the confidence of knowing that God is always in control.

Bible Verse: Isaiah 26:3- You keep him in perfect peace whose mind stays on you because he trusts in you.

Healthy: Take a few minutes to find out what fruit, herbs and vegetables are in season throughout the course of the year. When you know what is available then you can forage locally and pick and enjoy wild fruits, vegetables and herbs. You can also join a local foraging course, led by an expert, for more in-depth guidance. Forage for blackberries, raspberries, strawberries, cherries, elderberries and anything else that is native and local to you. It is free, most likely to be organic, fresh and an extremely delicious way to indulge yourself. There is nothing more gratifying than eating something that you have found and picked. Not to mention how great you will feel because not only have you actually picked your own fruit (better so if you can grow your own) but you have also spent some quality time in nature. If you have children, they will delight in a day out at a 'pick your own' farm! You can make jams, juices or preserves from the fruit you have collected.

Fit: The best body weight exercises like the plank and the push up can be varied so much that just doing these two exercises can be a full body workout in and of themselves. Challenge yourself to try and find as many variations and forms of these two exercises that work for your body type and enjoy how fit and strong you feel after a good and focused thirty-minute session.

When doing a plank, you should aim to hold the plank to at least 30 seconds squeezing your abdominals and gluteal muscles with each repetition.

The push up can be a challenging exercise for even the strongest of us. Start in full push up position and even if you can only lower yourself down a few centimetres and for one repetition at a time that is fine. Work from this point each time you do a push up and you will become stronger overtime. Remember to work until muscle failure to get the most out of each session.

Action: Push yourself a little harder. Acknowledge and relive your proudest moments in your life. Promise yourself that in everything, you will always do your very best! What is your next big goal? Write out what you need to do to accomplish this goal and get to work on making this goal a reality!

Day 17

Happy: Peace and quiet. It is in this stillness many of life's perplexities are simplified. Many a soul searched question answered and many a bitter gripe released.

Bible Verse: Proverbs 17: 27-28- The one who has knowledge uses words with restraint, and whoever has understanding is even-tempered. Even fools are thought wise if they keep silent, and discerning if they hold their tongues.

Healthy: Quinoa is a great wheat-free alternative to starchy grains. It belongs to the same family as beets, chard, and spinach and contains twice the protein content of rice or barley. Quinoa is a very good source of calcium, magnesium, and manganese, B vitamins, vitamin E and dietary fibre. Quinoa contains all nine essential amino acids making it a complete protein source.

To properly prepare quinoa, soak overnight in a glass bowl of water with the juice of a freshly squeezed lemon (one teaspoon of lemon juice to one cup of water) before cooking.

Once it has been cooked, quinoa can be eaten hot or cold, in salads, as the main entry or alone.

Fit: Quick, full body workouts are great for your training days when you are tired but still need to burn a few extra calories. When doing this sort of workout, make sure you are targeting whole body exercises. This shouldn't be a high intensity workout but one that focuses on strength, flexibility and utilises good breathing techniques. Think dynamic yoga or a functional flexibility type workout. Pre-plan your training schedule to ensure you are keeping your sleep and nutritional states on target and staying well hydrated in order to get the most out of these days! After this session which should last no more than an hour you should feel refreshed and invigorated.

Action: Schedule in some quiet time into your day each and every day. Set aside 15 minutes daily to be in silence and turn off the phone, radio, TV, laptop and anything that will distract you from your silent session. Listen to the sounds of nature, hear your heart beating, and come to terms with your breath. Listen, to the silence. Revel in how loud it actually is. Enjoy the peace and quiet. Do this often, your inner voice will thank you as you hone in on your ability to

hear it, listen to it and be at peace with it.

Day 18

Happy: Relaxation therapy is so immensely important to our overall health and wellbeing. Relaxation therapy is anything that completely and thoroughly relaxes you and puts you into almost a meditative state of inner calm and peace. It is different for us all.

For some, we find this state in nature (gardening, walks in the forests, woods, lakes), with animals, in reading, or writing, in creating, in a good film, in song or dance, in sport or in complete isolation. Find what works best for you and aim to make it a part of your lifestyle.

The benefits are a wholesome, balanced, calm, and centred person. It doesn't really get any better than that, except that you will feel totally and absolutely amazing so it is worth the effort to explore various forms until you find the one that works best for you!

Bible Verse: Isaiah 43:25-26 - I am He who blots out your transgressions for my own sake, and I will not remember your sins. Put me in remembrance; let us argue together; set forth your case, that you may be proved right.

Healthy: There is still a lot of controversy as to whether rice is considered a healthy food. Many cultures live and thrive off of rice-based diets, yet still there is still some controversy as to which rice is the healthier between the brown and white rice.

The difference between brown and white rice is that in milling, brown rice loses only a bit of the top layer above; the non-edible hull goes, but the bran and germ remain. White rice removes it all; the hull, awn, bran and berm are all gone, leaving behind the endosperm. Brown rice contains more nutrients than white rice but also has phytic acid and higher levels of arsenic. Brown rice also has a lower glycaemic index compared to white rice.

White rice is, however, easier to digest than brown rice. Many studies have shown that there are few overall differences, so eat the rice you like! As with all grains you should wash and soak the rice before cooking.

Again, everything in moderation and little is best, but if you are having rice enjoy it. If you can get organic rice (wild rice, red rice, black rice) even better, add a dollop of organic, grass-fed butter for a simply delicious dish.

Fit: Rebounding makes a splendid addition to your home gym as it boasts many physical and health benefits. It is a low impact form of exercise providing lymphatic drainage and boosting immune function.

Rebounding can help to increase bone mass, improve digestion and helps circulate oxygen throughout the body to increase energy. A rebounder is like a mini trampoline. It is lightweight and takes up very little space. It is a whole-body exercise system that improves muscle tone throughout the body and it is fun for grown-ups and children alike! Try rebounding for a few minutes each day.

Action: Remember those who have been good to you. Send a little present in the mail, a lovely greeting card or a simple thank you by text or a phone call. Let them know that you appreciate them and their kindness towards you, irrespective of how long ago it was. Every good deed deserves acknowledgement.

Day 19

Happy: Simple is best. It entails fewer complications, less drama, and minimal confusion. This motto can be applied to every area of life. In planning meals, simple and easy is best. In dress, simple and classy is best. In friends, simple and loving and drama free is best. In your home, simple and minimalistic is best and in your affairs simple and stress-free is best. Anything that causes unnecessary wanton worry means that somewhere somehow it can and needs to be simplified.

Bible Verse: Proverbs 13:7- A pretentious, showy life is an empty life; a plain and simple life is a full life.

Healthy: Steaming as opposed to frying and boiling your food is a much healthier option. Steam cooking retains the vitamins, minerals, and flavour of the food, keeps the food in its original form meaning that vegetables do not turn to mush, softens the fibres of the food and improves digestion. Steaming your food means that clean-up is easy as a variety of foods can be simultaneously cooked in the same unit.

Steaming your food is an energy efficient way to cook and can be done anywhere with an electricity supply.

If you are going on a self-catering holiday and need to cook healthily you can always take a steamer! You can steam anything from meat to legumes and of course vegetables. A sprinkle of tasty herbs and a dollop of grass-fed butter will make your meal extremely delicious.

Fit: Sprinting is a fantastic form of exercise and one of the key basic components in many sports. Sprinting is a great way to build muscle and burn fat. If you are pressed for time it is an excellent form of training. It is great for conditioning the heart and lungs and aside from increasing speed and power can also help to build physical endurance! You can add sprints into pretty much anything you do. Develop mental toughness as you push yourself to your limits!

Sprinting track workout: 10 by 200 m all out sprint repeats with 3-5 minutes rest in between each.

Sprinting park, pool or cycle workout: 10 by 30 second all out sprint repeats. Add a small incline for a further challenge. 2-3 minutes rest intervals in between each.

Warm up and cool down adequately before and after your sprint session!

Action: Stress reduction is imperative in maintaining balance in our day to day lives. Sometimes when we feel overwhelmed, we are unable to decipher the cause. Analyzing the different venues from which we can become stressed is crucial. Family, friends, home, work, bills, car, pets etc. are all potential causes. Look at how you can minimise and eliminate stress from your life and make a concerted effort to doing so consistently.

Day 20

Happy: Slow down. Take your time in life. Allow yourself to go through the processes and experiences of your time on earth free from the restraints of time. Slow down. Do not let time be a dictator to you. You are the creator, the maker, the boss and the dictator of your world. Live life on your terms and be free!

Bible Verse: 1 Corinthians 15:57- But thanks be to God! He gives us the victory through our Lord Jesus Christ.

Healthy: Teff is a wholesome, gluten free, delicious and healthy grain with a low glycaemic index (meaning your blood sugar levels are better regulated) that can be made into so many appetising dishes from cereals to snack bars to wraps and pancakes.

Teff is high in protein with a great combination of eight essential amino acids needed for the body's growth and repair. It has high amounts of calcium, manganese, phosphorous, iron, copper, aluminium, barium, thiamine, and vitamin C (which is not normally found in grains) and is low in sodium. The iron from teff is easily absorbed and is also recommended for people with low blood iron levels. It is highly fibrous which means that you feel fuller longer and also regulates your bowel movements.

Fit: Tae Bo created by the amazing Billy Banks is a total body fitness programme that integrates martial arts techniques such as kicks and punches in numerous high energy and exhilarating combinations. It is lively, result focused, highly inspiring and one of the best forms of exercise you can participate in to get and keep results. Billy Banks is motivating, committed and in each workout gives you his very best which means that after 30 minutes you are sweating, breathless and wanting more! And best of all, you see and feel the results!

Action: Tell someone close to you how much you really care for them and how much they really mean to you. Many times, we are fearful of 'wearing our hearts on our sleeves' and do not express to those who mean the most to us, our genuine love and care for them. Life is short and it is not guaranteed to any of us, so make your love known!

Day 21

Happy: If we continuously strive to understand the point of view of others, we have made an attempt at setting a firm and stable foundation for a relationship of openness, compromise, and empathy. We remove ego, and replace it instead with the wholeness of our being, love and pure kindness. It is in this space, that miracles can happen.

Bible Verse: Proverbs 4:7- The beginning of wisdom is this: Get wisdom. Though it cost all you have, get understanding.

Healthy: Unpasteurised dairy is essential to our health as it is rich in good bacteria. The bacteria found in raw dairy helps to enhance the levels of beneficial bacteria present in the gut. These bacterial allies are destroyed by pasteurisation and are absent in pasteurised and UHT milk. Raw dairy is also rich in natural vitamins and is very easy to digest! Raw dairy is not homogenised.

Homogenization is a process in which the fat molecules are broken up so there is no cream on top of the milk. This increases the likelihood of oxidation in the body which contributes to heart disease, hypertension (high blood pressure), and hyperlipidaemia (high cholesterol).

Further, raw and unpasteurized dairy from grass fed cows yields absolutely delicious, cream, yoghurt, butter and cheese in as close to their natural state and as full of as much goodness as they can contain as possible.

The best part of using raw dairy products is that usually the living conditions for the animals are better and animal welfare is adhered to.

Make sure you choose your dairy milk from a farm where animal welfare is a top priority and the animals are happy and content!

How to choose your milk:

Option One: Raw, organic milk from grass fed cows.

Option Two: Organic pasteurised, un-homogenized milk.

Option Three: Organic pasteurised, homogenised milk.

Option Four: Go dairy free: Hemp milk, almond milk, oat milk and coconut milk are fantastic. Opt for milk that is free from added oils, sugars and flavourings.

Option Five: Make your own milk from coconuts or sprouted nuts and seeds!

Fit: Want to take your training to another level? Add some uphill running. Find some steep hills, grab a towel, and a bottle of water and be prepared to work, and hard! Uphill running not only is an excellent way to shape and tone your body, especially the legs and buttock muscles, but it builds endurance, burns more calories and will increase your speed. Aim for 10 -12 hill repeats of 50-100m in length with an active recovery of a downhill jog. Run up, walk down. Enjoy a good stretch, a nutritionally dense meal, and a hot bath after to prevent the muscles from being overly sore the following day.

Action: Undertake a new hobby this month. Try something daring, something fun and something absolutely and totally exhilarating. Not sure where to start? Make a bucket list. Then choose an activity that you can do on a few occasions.

Example: **Bucket List**

Entry Number 1: Salsa dancing on a cruise ship in the Caribbean.

Preparation Hobby: Take one month of salsa lessons to learn how to salsa dance before the escapade! Have fun with it!

Remember that we only have one chance on planet earth, so we may as well enjoy our time here to the fullest.

Happy: Visualisation can help us to quickly accomplish a goal. It is so efficient because it permits us to first see (in our minds) the process(es) we need to go through, in addition, to feeling the accompanying emotions that we may experience in order to obtain our desired goal.

If you see it and believe it, you can achieve it.

Once you engage fully in this process by visualising situations as you would like them to be and committing to doing so continuously, you will see your visualisation become a reality.

Guided positive affirmations can also aid in enhancing your visualisations. To enhance your visualisations dwell in the feeling states of the end results of what you desire. If you desire wealth, how does it look and feel? If you desire love what does it look and feel like?

Take some time to find pictures of what you desire so that you can visualise them often. Place them somewhere that you can see though out the day.

Bible Verse: Matthew 5:8- Blessed are the pure in heart, for they shall see God.

Healthy: Apple cider vinegar has an incredible amount of health benefits and marvellously too can not only be consumed but can also be used around the home. It decreases bloating, enhances the vitamins and minerals in your food, can detox the body, can be used as a deodorizer, balances the PH of the blood and also can be used to clean fruits and vegetables, wash hair and as a mouth rinse. Amazing!

Fit: Volleyball is the perfect all-around sport. Play it at the park, on the beach or in the garden with children for a fun loving, full body and energising workout!

Action: For the next 40 days visualise yourself exactly where you want to be in the next five years. How will you get there? What you must do to accomplish this goal? What will it look like? How will it feel when you have accomplished your goals? Who will be on the journey with you? Take some time visualising this daily. Create a mood board with pictures of what the next five years will look like and sit and visualise daily until your desires become a reality.

Day 24

Happy: Worship is the complete and total surrender of our will to God's will. It is acknowledging His awesome power, His undeserved mercy, and His abounding grace. It is thanking Him for His unmerited favour and it is coming under His call and authority in and over our lives. We can worship all day, in song, in prayer, in action in thought in everything putting Him first and seeking him. It is here, that we find true bliss, pure joy and the deepest sense of fulfilment.

Bible Verse: Isiah 29:13- The Lord says: 'These people come near to me with their mouth and honour me with their lips, but their hearts are far from me. Their worship of me is based on merely human rules they have been taught'.

Healthy: Walnuts are considered to be the healthiest nut. They contain omega-3 fatty acids, which increase the activity of the brain. Walnuts have antioxidants and proteins that help in imparting a multitude of health benefits. Walnuts are also considered to be a 'power food' since they are believed to improve body stamina. Walnuts help to improve heart function, bone health, fight against cancer and boost mood. Add walnuts to salads, muesli, and yogurt or blend them into milk or nut butter. Simple and delicious!

Fit: Weightlifting should be undertaken by both men and women alike. Countless studies have debunked the myths that women weightlifting become overtly muscular and masculine. Contrary to the fact weightlifting can increase your metabolism, build muscle, prevent injury, increase flexibility and bone density, boost self-esteem, make you stronger and ward off depression.

If you don't know where to start, try a cross fit session for beginners, a body pump class or simply ask your gym instructor to carry you through the basics. Once you have an idea of what weightlifting exercises you enjoy the best include weight training into at least three of your sessions per week. Don't train the same muscles every session and make sure to stretch and cool down after a weight training session.

Action: Trade in worry for worship. Know that God is in control of everything! Pray, ask, believe you have received what you have asked for in prayer and then let it go. All is well.

Happy: Be proud of what you have accomplished in your life so far! Acknowledge the challenges, celebrate the good and learn from the bad. From within the deepest yearnings of your heart, go forth in zeal and do what makes you happy, chase after what makes you smile and live in perfect and abundant peace.

Bible Verse: John 15:7- If you abide in me, and my words abide in you, ask whatever you wish, and it will be done for you.

Healthy: Commit to eating the best you possibly can. Where possible opt for raw, organic, pesticide and GMO-free foods, grass fed and pasture raised meats, milks and butter, fermented foods, sprouted foods and grains, bone broths, fresh juices and beverages such as kimchi and kefir. Try new foods and aim to try a new fruit or vegetable per week. Explore the foods of different cultures adding the ones that you like to your diet. Enjoy what you eat.

Fit: Commit to moving every day! Do something. Don't over commit and underachieve. Set a realistic standard and maintain that standard every day. Enjoy the process. It's fun!

Action: Live, Laugh, Love!

Well done! You've made it to the end. At this point you should have discovered along the way, the things that help you to be balanced physically, nutritionally and spiritually. Hopefully you have developed the ideal routine to help you live a wholesome and healthy life. Remember, this is just the beginning. Continue to learn and grow.

Notes

Notes

Notes

Notes

Go forth in good health, be in peace and live your life within
your purpose!

May it always be well with you!

www.ingramcontent.com/pod-product-compliance
Lightning Source LLC
Chambersburg PA
CBHW061713250726
48657CB00002B/607